Toward a Containment Strategy for Smallpox Bioterror

An Individual-Based Computational Approach

Joshua M. Epstein, Derek A. T. Cummings,
Shubha Chakravarty, Ramesh M. Singa, and
Donald S. Burke

BROOKINGS INSTITUTION PRESS

Washington, D.C.

Copyright © 2004

THE BROOKINGS INSTITUTION

1775 Massachusetts Avenue, N.W., Washington, D.C. 20036
www.brookings.edu

Library of Congress Cataloging-in-Publication data
Toward a containment strategy for smallpox bioterror : an individual-based computational approach /
Joshua M. Epstein…[et al.].
    p. ; cm.
    Includes bibliographical references and index.
    ISBN 0-8157-2455-1 (pbk. : alk. paper)
    1. Smallpox—Epidemiology—Computer simulation. 2. Bioterrorism—Computer simulation.
3. Epidemics—Prevention—Computer simulation.
    [DNLM: 1. Smallpox—prevention & control—United States. 2. Bioterrorism—United States.
3. Communicable Disease Control—United States. 4. Computer Simulation—United States. 5. Smallpox
Vaccine—therapeutic use—United States. WC 588 T737 2004] I. Epstein, Joshua M., 1951– II. Title.
    RA644.S6T69 2004
    614.5'21'0113—dc22   2004004249

9 8 7 6 5 4 3 2 1

The paper used in this publication meets minimum requirements of the
American National Standard for Information Sciences—Permanence of Paper for
Printed Library Materials: ANSI Z39.48-1992.

Typeset in Adobe Garamond

Design and composition by Circle Graphics
Columbia, Maryland

Printed by Phoenix Color
Rockaway, New Jersey

Contents

Acknowledgments

This research was funded by a grant from the Alfred P. Sloan Foundation. For helpful discussion, the authors thank Ellis McKenzie, Edward Kaplan, James Koopman, Jon Parker, Nancy Gallagher, Elisa Harris, and John Steinbruner.

Introduction

Since the September 11, 2001, terrorist attacks in New York and Washington and the subsequent anthrax outbreaks on the east coast of the United States, bioterror concerns have focused on smallpox. Routine smallpox vaccinations in the United States ended in 1972. The level of immunity remaining from these earlier vaccinations is uncertain but is assumed to be degraded substantially. For present modeling purposes, we assume it to be nil.

As a weapon, smallpox would be very different from anthrax. Anthrax is not a communicable disease. Smallpox is highly communicable. With a case fatality rate of roughly 30 percent (meaning that 30 percent of infected individuals die), it is also very deadly. Many of those who survive the disease, furthermore, are permanently disfigured, their well-being compromised for life.

There is now heated debate on the appropriate national strategy for smallpox bioterror.[1] Who should be vaccinated?

---

1. In the summer of 2001, researchers at the Johns Hopkins Center for Civilian Biodefense Strategies, in collaboration with several other organizations, formulated a policy exercise known as Dark Winter, which raised many important questions for bioterror attack response; see O'Toole, Mair, and Inglesby (2002).

Everyone who volunteers? Targeted subpopulations? When should immunization begin? Immediately? Only after a confirmed attack? What is the role of quarantine?

In this monograph, we present a county-level individual-based computational model of a smallpox epidemic.[2] We review and criticize the two main vaccination strategies currently under discussion: trace and mass vaccination. Based on the model, we then develop a distinct "hybrid" strategy that differs sharply from both, while combining useful aspects of each. It involves both preemptive (that is, pre-release) and reactive measures. As the basis for a national smallpox containment strategy, we believe it offers important advantages over the alternatives.

MODELS

In gauging the scale of a smallpox bioterror threat, and in designing an effective policy response, it is crucial to have *epidemic models* depicting the spatial spread of the disease in a relevant setting. Without the use of explicit models, there is no systematic way to gauge uncertainty or to evaluate competing intervention strategies. Building on previous work, we have developed an individual-based computational modeling environment for the study of epidemic dynamics in general (see appendix A).[3] This can be

---

2. Individual-based modeling is also called agent-based modeling. To avoid confusion between our agents (individual people) and infectious disease agents, we use the term individual-based modeling predominantly.

3. See Burke (1998); Grefenstette and others (1997); Burke and others (1998); Epstein and Axtell (1996); Epstein (1997).

applied to an indefinite variety of pathogens and social structures. Here, we develop an individual-based model of smallpox at the county level (an application to genetically modified smallpox is also noted).[4]

In contrast to compartmental epidemic models, which assume perfect homogeneous mixing and mass action kinetics,[5] the individual-based approach explicitly tracks the progression of the disease through *each individual* (thus populations become highly heterogeneous by health status during simulations) and tracks the contacts of each individual with others in relevant social networks and geographical areas (for example, family members, co-workers, schoolmates). All rules for individual agent movement (for example, to and from workplace, school, and hospital) and for contacts with and transmissions to other people are explicit, as is stochasticity (for example, in contacts). No homogeneous mixing assumptions are employed at any level. The prime social units that loom largest in the smallpox data,[6] such as hospitals and families, are explicitly represented, and our vaccination (and isolation) strategy is focused on these units of social structure. Calibration of our model to these data, and statistical analysis of core model runs, are discussed below.

Our model differs from the primary (and valuable) competing approaches, in a number of ways. For example,

---

4. For an introduction to the individual-based modeling technique, see Epstein and Axtell (1996). For diverse applications of the methodology, see Brian and others (2002).

5. Anderson and May (1991); Kaplan, Craft, and Wein (2002).

6. Mack (1972).

it differs from that of Halloran and coauthors in its explicit inclusion of hospitals. Most fundamentally, as a "pure" individual-based model, it eschews all homogeneous mixing assumptions at any level, in contrast to the models of both Halloran and coauthors and Kaplan, Craft, and Wein.[7]

7. Halloran and others (2002); Kaplan, Craft, and Wein (2002). There are further differences, including parametric ones. For useful remarks comparing continuous and discrete individual approaches in the present connection, see Koopman (2002).

The County-Level Model

The software we have developed permits generalization to multiple levels of social structure. For present purposes, we model a county composed of towns, hospitals, households, schools, and workplaces.

STRUCTURE AND CALIBRATION

The model structure was chosen for comparability to historical data describing the relationship between smallpox cases and the individuals who transmitted the disease to those cases in forty-nine outbreaks of smallpox in Europe from 1950 to 1971. This data set reveals the crucial role of hospital and household transmission in smallpox outbreaks. We wished to build the simplest model that captured the heterogeneity of transmission in the different settings of hospitals, families, workplaces, and schools. To ensure the replicability of our results, numerical assumptions and technical details are given in appendix A. Selected salient assumptions are noted in the text.

The model parameters governing the probability of transmission per contact and the contact rates in different social settings were chosen through a calibration of simulated epidemics with the historical data. As noted above, these data describe outbreaks resulting from forty-nine importations of a single case of smallpox into nonendemic Europe during the period 1950–71.[8] Two distributions from these data were used for the calibration: the distribution of the number of cases resulting from each of these importations and the distribution describing the proportion of cases resulting from exposure in a hospital setting, in a workplace or school setting, and in the home. A combinatorial sweep of the core parameters—the per contact transmission probability and the contact rates in the hospital, the home, and the workplace or school—was performed and the distribution of these results over many simulation runs was compared to the historical data. In all, approximately 10,000 runs were performed. The parameters that minimized the sum of squared deviations from the two historical distributions were chosen.

In the present version of the general model, each town is assumed to contain 100 family households, each with two working adults and two school-aged children—400 individuals in total. With two towns, the county population is thus 800.

Each town has one school and one workplace. All children attend their own town's school (there is no intertown busing). A small fraction of adults, by contrast, do commute to work in the other town. In our base runs, we assume that 10 percent of adults commute. There is a single county hospital, used by both towns. A small number of adults (in the present version, five) from each town work in the common hospital. Finally, there is a single morgue housing all individuals who have died.

---

8. Mack (1972).

TIME AND CONTACTS

Each modeling day is equally divided between a "daytime," when adults work and children attend school, and a "nighttime," when family members (exclusively) interact at home. Each of these phases of the day is composed of several rounds, in which each individual is processed, or "activated," once. The essential event that occurs when an individual is active is contact with other individuals. In our model, the active individual is contacted by randomly selected individuals from the relevant pool (family members or immediate neighbors at work or school). Numerical assumptions regarding contacts and transmissions per contact are given in appendix A. Note that the per contact probability of contracting the infection depends on the stage of illness the contacting individual is in.

GRAPHICS

The graphical setup is depicted in figure 1, which shows two snapshots of the county, labeled nighttime and daytime. Two towns can be seen, Circletown and Squaretown, inhabited respectively by circle individuals and square individuals. (Circles and squares are used simply to make commuting individuals discernible and to depict the hospital workers' hometowns.) As runs progress, individuals return home at night and go to work and school during the day, a process that iterates indefinitely. That summarizes the social contact process. Meanwhile, the epidemic is running its course.

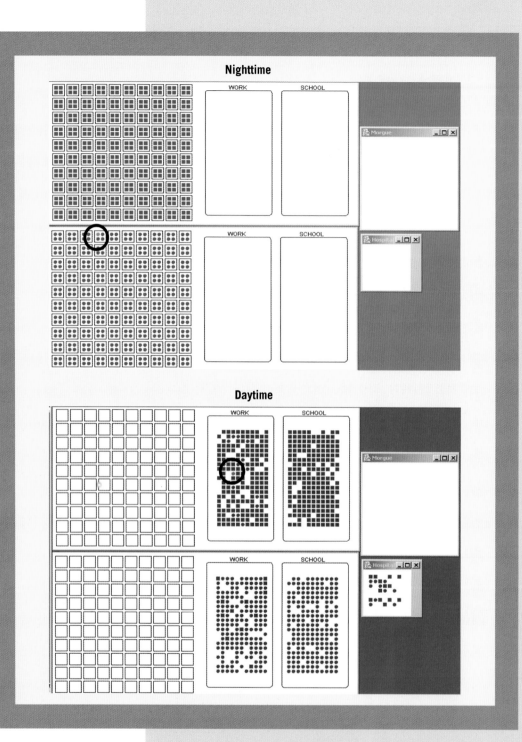

FIGURE 1
County View: Night and Day

Note: An illustrative commuter is colored green and circled.

SMALLPOX ASSUMPTIONS

Our assumptions about the natural history of smallpox in the individual are illustrated by the timeline in figure 2, which also describes the color coding used in the model graphics. Before we release our index case—the first infective individual—into the population, we assume all individuals to be susceptible; that is, we assume no background of immunity (for example, from previous vaccinations). Susceptible individuals are colored blue. Referring to the timeline, let us assume an individual contracts the infection at day 0. At that point, she/he is colored green. Although the person is infected with smallpox, she/he is asymptomatic and noncontagious for twelve days. However, unless the infected individual is vaccinated within four days of exposure, the vaccine is ineffective. As a policy matter, this is a critical point: it will be necessary to vaccinate infected

FIGURE 2
Progression of Smallpox

Source: Fenner and others (1988).

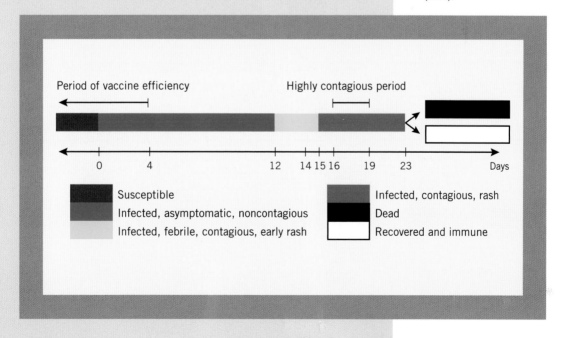

people *before* they manifest any symptoms. From day 12 to day 15, infected individuals are assumed to be febrile and contagious (infectious) with smallpox, but do not yet exhibit the smallpox rash. They feel sick, but precise diagnosis is not yet possible.

At the end of day 15, smallpox rash is finally evident. After twelve hours in this state, individuals are assumed to be hospitalized. After eight more days (day 23 of illness), during which they have a cumulative 30 percent probability of mortality, surviving individuals recover and return to circulation permanently immune to further infection. Dead individuals are colored black and placed in the morgue.[9] Immune individuals are colored white. Contagiousness varies in the course of the infection. Individuals are assumed to be 2 times as infectious during days 16 through 19 as during days 12 through 15. In the final phases of the rash, infectivity returns to the day 12 value, as indicated in figure 2. In the simulated epidemics below, individuals will be colored by their state: healthy (blue), infected (green), contagious early rash (yellow), rash (red), dead (black), or immune (white). At any time, the population will be heterogeneous by health status.

---

9. The morgue is a closed system, so no transmission occurs there.

Simulated Epidemics

3

We present a number of runs and statistical analyses. All simulations in this paper assume a single initial infective individual (for example, a bioterrorist or bioterror victim), who is an adult commuter.[10]

We present snapshots from our computer simulation. It is important to note, when presenting a simulated epidemic, that any such realization is but one sample path of a stochastic process. There are run-to-run differences due to random effects, even when all parameters are fixed across runs. Indeed, as we shall see, these random effects can be dramatic, spelling the difference between large-scale epidemics and abortive ones. Hence, a statistical treatment is necessary and is offered below. To begin, however, it builds intuition to "watch" the base case epidemic unfold in our county over time. Again, we imagine a smallpox bioterrorist initiating the epidemic by infecting (or by being) a commuting adult.

---

10. On reflection, the assumption of a single index case is quite conservative. In a city of 12 million (such as Manhattan), one initial infective per 800 would translate into 15,000 initial infectives. Of course, this assumes a *linear* scale-up, which may well be unrealistic. Our point is simply that, scaled in any plausible way, one in 800 will translate into an enormous attack force in the bioterror interpretation. Although we do not believe we are artificially simplifying the problem, our software allows for expansion by orders of magnitude, as discussed below.

BASE CASE: NO INTERVENTION

The base case scenario is obtained by setting model parameters to values found by calibration to the European data set and by assuming no preexisting immunity in the population. The epidemic is allowed to simply run its course, without any vaccination or isolation strategy. Figure 3 presents nine frames (snapshots) from the full simulation, which can be viewed as a movie at www.brookings.edu/es/dynamics/models/bioterrorism.htm.

Frame 1 simply shows our index case, a Circletown commuter, at home at night. He is green, indicating that he is infected but asymptomatic. Frame 2 shows the index case at his Squaretown workplace the next day. Frame 3 depicts the situation on day 15, at which point our index case has developed the full smallpox rash. Notice that by this point, he has spread the disease to others (colored green), but none of them are aware that they are ill, a situation that persists into day 16 (frame 4), when the index reports to the hospital. In this particular run, he dies eight days later and is taken to the morgue on day 24, as shown in frame 5. No one else in the county yet realizes that he or she is sick. Frame 6 depicts the situation at day 42. Notice that the epidemic is now far worse in Squaretown than in Circletown, despite the fact that it began in Circletown. So, seemingly sensible strategies like "concentrate vaccination on the town where the outbreak begins" may do poorly. By the time one vaccinates there, the epidemic may well have spread beyond. Frame 7 (day 52) and frame 8 (day 62) show the hospital filling to capacity and the morgue filling up. They also show that many people recover (colored white). Finally, the epidemic's

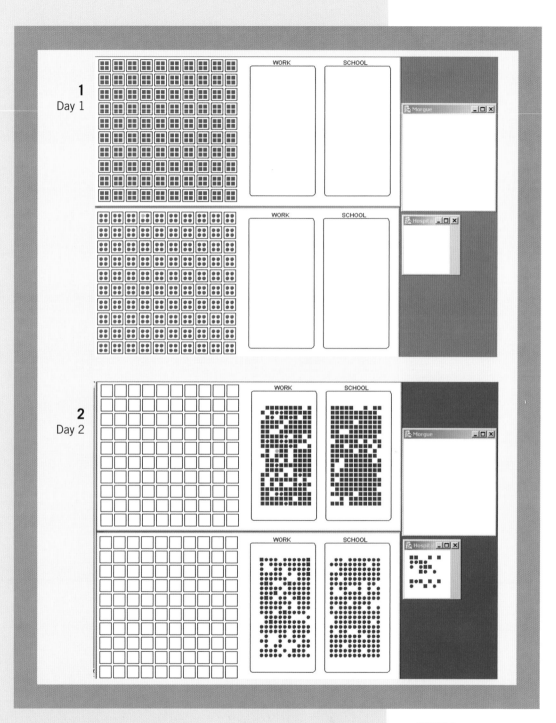

FIGURE 3
Base Case Run:
No Interventions

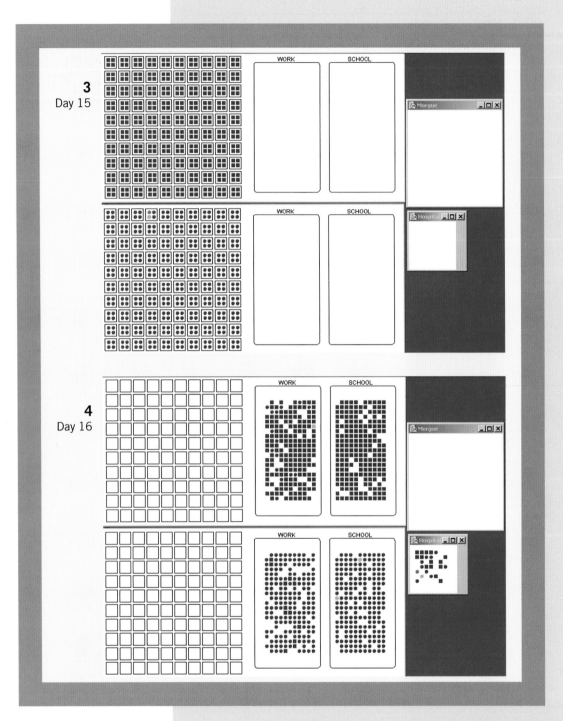

FIGURE 3
(*Continued*)

14

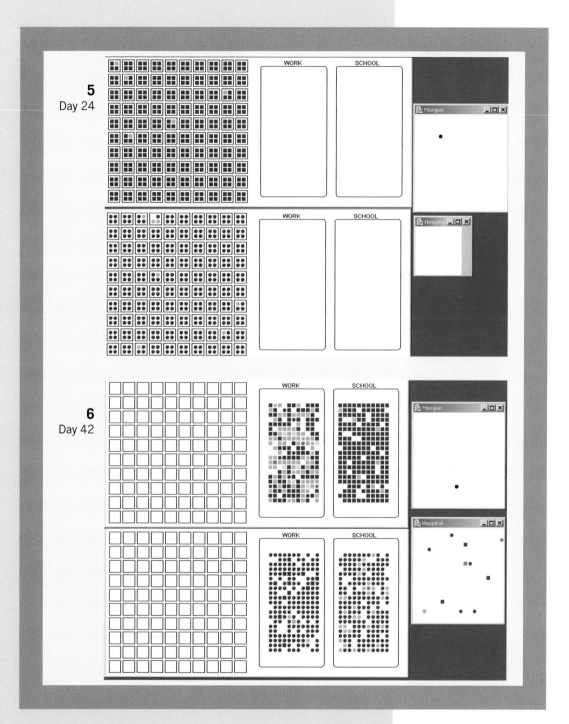

FIGURE 3
(*Continued*)

15

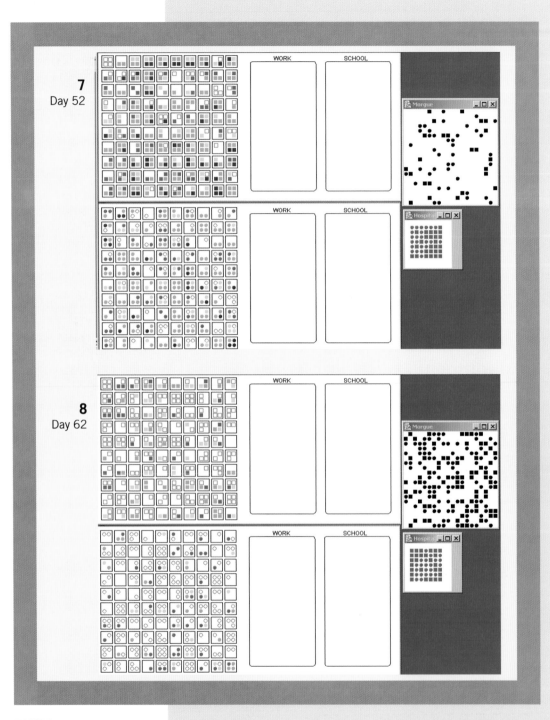

FIGURE 3
(*Continued*)

16

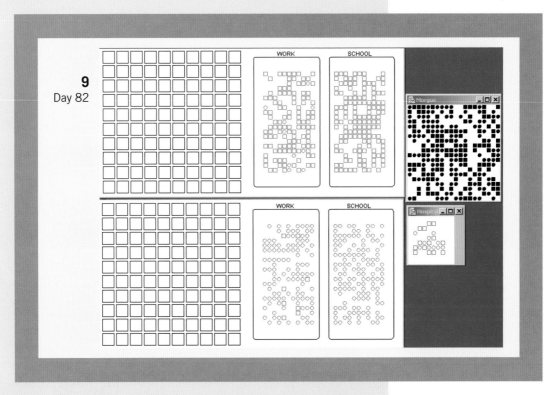

FIGURE 3
(*Continued*)

end state is shown in frame 9 (day 82). With no intervention, everyone in the county eventually contracts smallpox, and roughly 30 percent die of the disease.[11] It is noteworthy that the base case assumes no background of immunity. It may represent well the dynamics when European smallpox was first introduced into virgin indigenous populations.

Figure 4 shows typical time series of incidence (top panel) and number of infected individuals (bottom panel) for a representative simulation in which there is no intervention.

---

11. Here, we assume that agents continue to go to work and school, that hospitalized individuals are not isolated, and that no agents flee the county.

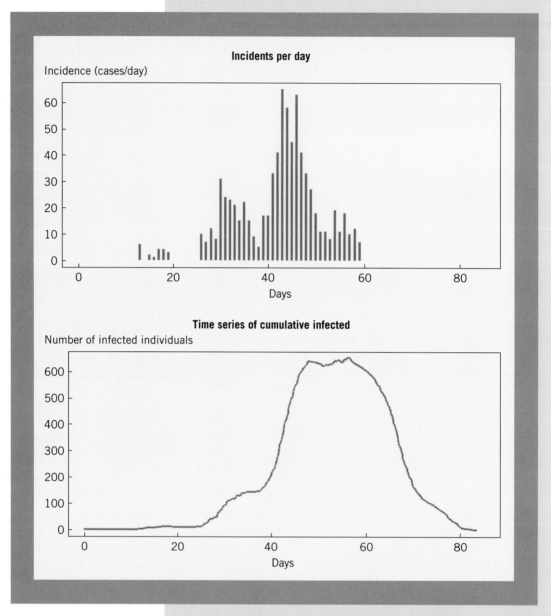

FIGURE 4
Typical Results for Base
Case Run

This, then, is the problem we wish to address. What is the appropriate policy response? We begin with a review of traditional vaccination strategies and their problems. We then offer a hybrid vaccination strategy of our own. The substantial role of voluntarism is noted.

Vaccination Strategies

4

The vaccination strategies that have loomed largest in the policy debate thus far are trace vaccination and mass vaccination. Each has advantages and disadvantages.

TRACE VACCINATION

Trace vaccination is an elegant idea. Given a confirmed smallpox case, one traces every contact the individual has had and vaccinates that group. The Centers for Disease Control has adopted priority-based trace vaccination in its Smallpox Response Plan and Guidelines,[12] discussed more fully in appendix B. Contacts are technically defined as "persons who had . . . close proximity contact (< 2 meters = 6.5 feet) with a confirmed or suspected smallpox patient after the onset of the smallpox patient's fever."

This approach was effectively used in the worldwide smallpox eradication effort.[13] However, there is great concern that in advanced industrial settings, an individual's network of contacts is huge. It will include persons who rode the same

12. U.S. Centers for Disease Control, "Smallpox Response Plan and Guidelines" (version 3.0), www.bt.cdc.gov/agents/smallpox/response-plan/ [accessed December 5, 2002].

13. Fenner and others (1988).

urban metro system or flew out of the same airport, and thus contacts will be dispersed all over the city or country. The resource demands for full trace vaccination quickly become daunting. The value of incomplete, or imperfect, trace vaccination has not received sufficient attention. Below, we present a new strategy involving such an approach.

MASS VACCINATION

Indiscriminate mass vaccination poses a distinct set of problems. The first is that administration of the smallpox vaccine is not without risk. Complications from the vaccine include postvaccinal encephalitis, progressive vaccinia, eczema vaccinatum, generalized vaccinia, and accidental infection. It is estimated that forty complications would result from every 1 million doses given. Of these, an estimated one in every 1 million persons vaccinated would die from complications.[14]

Second, vaccination is not recommended for a significant proportion of the population—groups at special risk of vaccine complications. These groups include persons with eczema; patients undergoing chemotherapy for leukemia, lymphoma, or generalized malignancy; patients with HIV; persons with hereditary immune deficiencies; and pregnant women.[15] Vaccination of these persons, or even inadvertent inoculation with the vaccine strain, could lead to serious disease or death.

In summary, while perfect trace vaccination is infeasible from a practical standpoint, mass vaccination carries

---

14. Lane and others (1969).
15. Henderson and others (1999).

relatively greater risks of vaccine-related morbidity and mortality.

THE POLICY CHALLENGE

The challenge for government is therefore as follows: *Design a policy that is more feasible than trace vaccination, less risky than mass vaccination, and highly effective in containing a smallpox epidemic.* In designing such a policy, we exploit the essential feature of epidemics as dynamic processes: they are nonlinear stochastic phenomena.

Bifurcation and Epidemic Quenching

5

Epidemiologists have long known that introductions of disease into populations with some background level of immunity can yield large outbreaks or outbreaks of just a handful of cases, with no outbreaks of sizes between the very small and the very large. This bifurcation phenomenon is described in the literature by the results of stochastic compartmental models, using the terms *stochastic extinction* or *fade-out*.[16] We introduce the term *epidemic quenching* to denote dynamics in which the stochastic extinction occurs at the scale of discrete social units. Thus, introductions can be quenched at the level of the family, the workplace, or the town. We believe this approach accurately captures the local stochastic nature of real epidemics. The best vaccination strategies may well be those that take advantage of the importance of social structure to real epidemics. What strategies might give the public a reasonable chance that an epidemic will be "quenched"?

The actual data on European introductions of smallpox from 1950 to 1971 are shown in figure 5. This data set is focused on the question, where did infected individuals contract smallpox? Importantly, 50 percent contracted it at the

16. Anderson and May (1991); Bailey (1953); Whittle (1955).

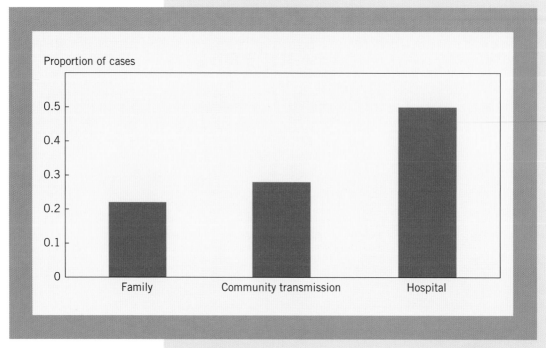

Proportion of cases

FIGURE 5
Smallpox Cases, by
Relationship to Transmitting
Case, Europe 1950–71

Source: Mack (1972).
Note: Sample includes 680
cases.

hospital and 22 percent contracted it from family. The remaining community transmission (28 percent) resulted primarily from workplace, school, and casual contacts.[17] Our model was built with these units of social structure in mind, and includes hospitals, families, work, and other venues precisely to allow calibration to these data. As discussed above, we have fit the model to these data. A strength of the agent-based approach is that it facilitates a focus on heterogeneous social units with distinctive internal dynamics, in contrast to models with homogeneous compartments.

These European smallpox epidemic data clearly suggest that vaccinating hospital workers preemptively (before an attack) and vaccinating family contacts reactively (as soon as

---

17. These data exclude fomite transmissions and include some undetermined and unreported transmissions.

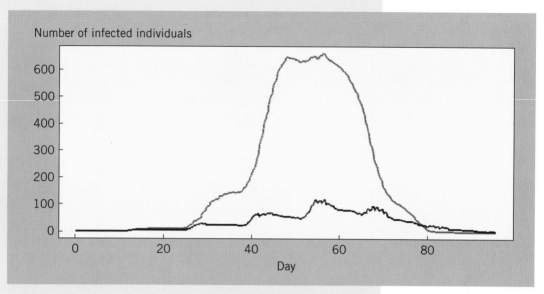

Number of infected individuals

FIGURE 6
Results of Interventions

Note: The black time series shows a typical run that implements our suggested interventions. The red time series is the original curve from figure 4, which shows the no-intervention case.

possible afterward) would be a powerful defense. Figure 6 indicates that this is, in fact, the case. The red curve is the time series for a typical run with no interventions. The black curve is the time series for the strategy just stated: preemptive hospital vaccination, isolation of cases in the hospital, and reactive contact tracing of household members of cases. Notice that none of these measures involves elaborate contact tracing. If, to these measures, we begin to add moderate levels of mass preemptive vaccination, a significant fraction of epidemics are quenched in our model.

QUENCHING THROUGH COMBINED VACCINATION EFFORTS

Combining vaccination efforts—preemptive mass vaccination, preemptive vaccination of hospital workers, and reactive household trace vaccination—has dramatic effects on both the quenching (confinement of the disease to discrete social units) and the extent (absolute number of cases) of the epidemic. Since epidemics are stochastic, single runs can be misleading. Therefore, we conducted a statistical analysis. We assume that all hospital workers in the model are vaccinated preemptively. Then, for five distinct levels of reactive family trace vaccination (0, 25, 50, 75, and 100 percent), we study how the course of the epidemic varies as we increase the level of preemptive mass vaccination. At each level of mass vaccination, the model was run 100 times, with a different random seed each run. The number infected in each run is plotted in red.

The entire analysis is shown in figure 7. The main observation is that with increasing levels of family contact tracing, the distribution of the number infected in each epidemic shifts downward at every level of preemptive mass vaccination.

While the best policy results are obtained at 100 percent family contact tracing (panel 7e), the most illuminating scientific results are evident in panel 7d, which displays 75 percent family contact tracing. Here, we see clear bifurcations: particularly at lower levels of preemptive mass vaccination (50 percent or less) the addition of reactive family contact tracing produces a trimodal distribution of epidemics. We examine this 75 percent family contact tracing case in much greater detail in figure 8. This offers a higher resolution version of panel 7d, with the frequency explicitly plotted above each point.

We believe that the bifurcations seen in figures 7 and 8 are clear evidence of quenching at the level of structural social units. We are studying this phenomenon in greater depth.

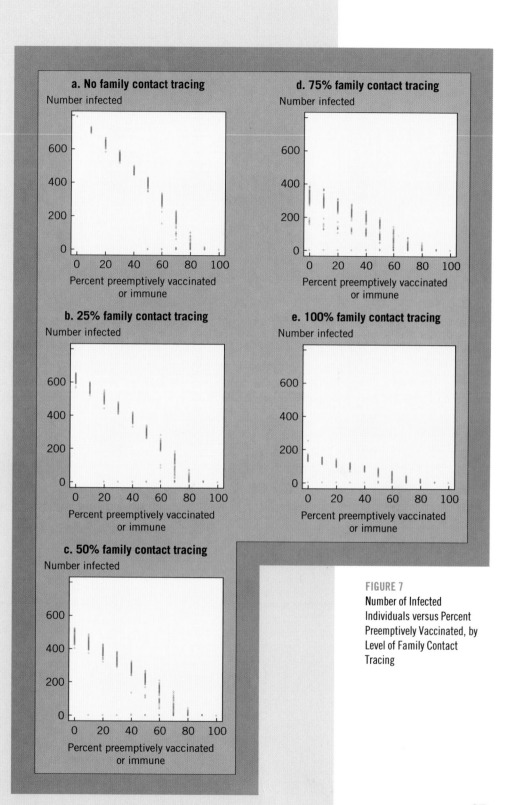

FIGURE 7
Number of Infected Individuals versus Percent Preemptively Vaccinated, by Level of Family Contact Tracing

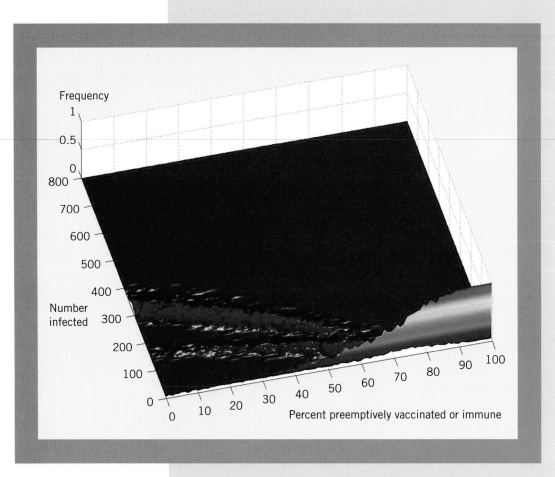

FIGURE 8
Probability Surface of the
75 Percent Family Contact
Tracing Case

A Balanced
Policy

6

As noted, the best *policy* results are obtained at 100 percent reactive family contact tracing, shown in figure 7, panel e. Figure 9 shows the cumulative distribution of infection for the 60 percent preemptive mass vaccination level in that panel (7e). We cite this level of preemptive vaccination because it is obtainable at minimum risk, by revaccinating those individuals successfully vaccinated in the past.[18] This group is highly unlikely to suffer any of the side effects emphasized above.

The vertical axis of figure 9 is the frequency of simulated outbreaks (for $n = 100$) that result in fewer than the number of infections indicted on the x-axis. So, for example, 100 percent of the simulation runs result in fewer than seventy infections (twenty-one deaths).

Now, what one sees reported in the media is, in a sense, the easy part of the policy problem. If there is a confirmed bioterror release of smallpox, the government must, of course, provide vaccine. Politically, there is no alternative. Hence the U.S. government is stockpiling 286 million doses.[19] But the deeper and politically tougher question is what to do *before* any release to contain the epidemic and ease

---

18. U.S. Bureau of the Census, 2000 Summary File, www.census.gov/census2000/states/us.html [accessed December 5, 2002].

19. Kaplan, Craft, and Wein (2002).

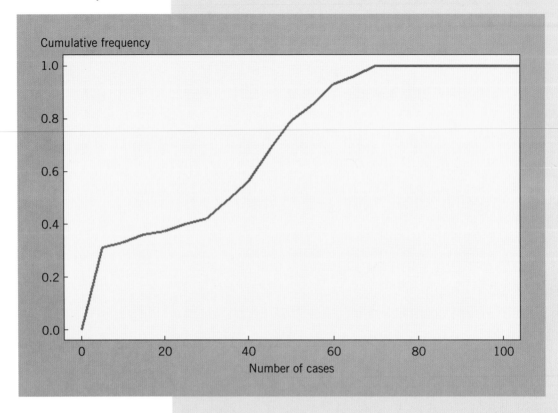

FIGURE 9
Cumulative Distribution of
Outcomes for the Case of
100 Percent Family Contact
Tracing and Preemptive
Hospital Vaccination and
60 Percent Preemptive Mass
Vaccination

the burden of further vaccination if necessary (and the atten-dant risks of indiscriminate immunizations). In our two-town county model, the following mix of preemptive and reactive policy measures achieves these goals:

Preemptive
  1. Vaccination of 100 percent of hospital workers
  2. Voluntary revaccination of healthy vaccinees (indi-viduals successfully vaccinated in the past)

Reactive
  3. Isolation in hospital of confirmed cases
  4. Vaccination of household members of confirmed cases

Referring to figure 9, under this package, 100 percent of the simulated outbreaks result in fewer than seventy cases (twenty-one deaths), 75 percent of outbreaks yield fewer than forty-five cases (fourteen deaths), and 50 percent of outbreaks yield fewer than thirty-five cases (eleven deaths). This certainly qualifies as *containment* compared to the no-intervention base case, in which the entire population of 800 individuals becomes infected and roughly 240 die in virtually all runs.

In our model, this package of measures offers the public an excellent chance that a bioterror smallpox attack will be quenched and limited in its severity and sharply reduces the logistical burden and public health risk of further vaccination if necessary. In particular, it minimizes the risks of indiscriminate mass vaccination and, in contrast to complete trace vaccination, is entirely feasible. Given a credible bioterrorist threat,[20] this combination of measures can serve as the basis for a smallpox containment strategy.

---

20. The credibility of such a threat at this time is a topic that lies outside the bounds of this research.

Research Conducted under the Auspices of the Smallpox Modeling Working Group

7

Since the completion of the above research, the Brookings-Hopkins team has joined the Smallpox Modeling Working Group of the Secretary's Advisory Council on Public Health Preparedness of the Department of Health and Human Services. This working group was established and is chaired by D. A. Henderson, who also chairs the advisory council. One of the working group's major undertakings was to collectively agree on core model parameters, distributions, and behavioral assumptions. The following major model extensions were then assigned and have since been made.

—Expand the population from 800 to 6,000 and 50,000 agents

—Expand the range of bioterror attacks from the single initial infective to 10 initial infectives in the 6,000 agent case, and to 500 initial infectives (for example, an aerosol release in a movie theater) in the 50,000 agent case

—Explore social structures beyond the original two-town setup, including a ring of towns and a hub-and-spoke arrangement of towns

—Beyond ordinary smallpox, model modified (by background immunity) and hemorrhagic smallpox

—Use full distributions for the incubation periods and infectiousness of smallpox, rather than the step functions of the original model (arriving at agreed assumptions for the natural history of the disease in humans consumed a number of working group meetings)

—Use explicit assumptions about when smallpox cases would be recognized in the hospital (interventions start once the first case is recognized)

—Vary the care-seeking behavior of individuals based upon the type of smallpox they contract (for example, hemorrhagic cases seek care almost immediately after the onset of symptoms, whereas modified cases have some chance of not reporting to the hospital for three days after the onset of symptoms)

—Model ten different intervention scenarios, from preemptive vaccination of hospital workers only (various percentage levels) to surveillance and containment to varying levels of postattack voluntary mass vaccination, and combinations of these.

All of these extensions and results are presented in the report "Individual-based Computational Modeling of Smallpox Epidemic Control Strategies."[21] While the scenarios that were assigned the working group for analysis differed from the one treated above, none of the analyses in that report challenge the fundamental soundness of the containment approach developed in the present monograph.

---

21. Burke and others (2004); to be published.

Further
Research

8

We plan to deepen our analysis of smallpox proper, extend our study of interventions, and examine a number of further topics.

EXPANDING SCALE

Regarding smallpox proper, further sensitivity analyses will be worthwhile. First among them, perhaps, is the question of scale-up. Do our fundamental results change when we expand the model to populations orders of magnitude larger? We plan to scale the model up to 1.7 million individuals. Other worthwhile sensitivity analyses would further vary the number of initial cases and the patterns and levels of commuting, for example.

VACCINATING CONTACTS OF CONTACTS

Current modeling efforts (including ours) assess trace vaccination efforts assuming that these entail only the identification and vaccination of contacts of confirmed infected individuals. They have not assessed the effects of vaccinating contacts of contacts of confirmed infected individuals. The Centers for Disease Control's Smallpox Response and Guidelines and the worldwide smallpox eradication effort both cite the importance of vaccinating contacts of contacts in containing smallpox outbreaks.[22] Our modeling effort has built the capability to quantitatively assess the impact of such an approach, and this will be the subject of further inquiry.

SEASONALITY

Smallpox epidemic dynamics are known to vary with the seasons. Spread efficiency increases in winter relative to summer. These seasonal variations could affect the appropriate mix of intervention strategies. Seasonality, then, is another promising area of further research.

FAMILY ISOLATION

Beyond vaccination, isolation is another policy. One can imagine "trace isolation," in which the dendrite of a confirmed smallpox carrier's contacts is traced and isolated. But this is as intractable as trace vaccination. One can also imagine broad isolation strategies, like closing all schools and workplaces or banning cross-town traffic (essentially quarantine of entire towns).

More discriminating than quarantine but less demanding than trace isolation is the following strategy, which we term *family isolation*: if any member of a household is diagnosed (presumably at the hospital) to have smallpox, all other household members stay home. This is surprisingly effective

22. U.S. Centers for Disease Control, "Smallpox Response Plan and Guidelines" (version 3.0), www.bt.cdc.gov/agents/smallpox/response-plan/ [accessed December 5, 2002]; Fenner and others (1988).

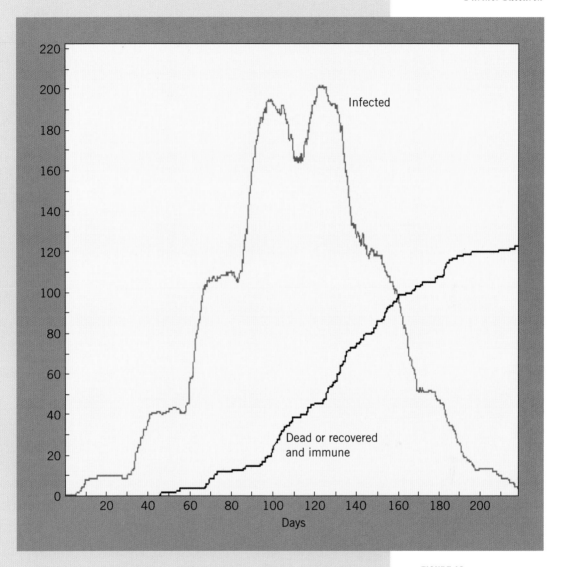

FIGURE 10
Typical Time Series for
Household Isolation Only

on its own. Indeed, as figure 10 suggests, with no vaccination or other additional interventions, this strategy is roughly as effective as random vaccination of half the population.

This makes the important methodological point that epidemics involve two dynamics. The first, the course of the disease in the individual, is biomedical. The second, the spatial contact process among individuals, is social. Our family

37

isolation policy operates only on the social contact process, but would be a surprisingly powerful adjunct to the vaccination strategies articulated earlier. Isolation is particularly relevant to SARS (Severe Acute Respiratory Syndrome), for which no vaccine is available. Further voluntary measures worthy of analysis are the use of masks, gloves, and other individual protective options. Among topics beyond smallpox, the threat of novel pathogens looms large.

NOVEL PATHOGENS: IL-4 SMALLPOX

In the wake of the recent Australian mousepox incident, there has been concern that incorporation of the interleukin-4 gene into smallpox would produce a more deadly pathogen that we have termed IL-4 smallpox.[23] Precisely how IL-4 smallpox would behave in human hosts is uncertain, but it is known that "interleukin-4 mediates downregulation of antiviral cytokine expression and cytotoxic T-lymphocyte responses and exacerbates vaccinia virus infection in vivo."[24] As a consequence, it is plausible that the pathogenicity (unvaccinated fatality rate) of IL-4 smallpox would substantially exceed that of unadulterated smallpox, that the smallpox vaccine would be considerably less effective against IL-4 smallpox than against smallpox, and that the transmissibilities of IL-4 and unmodified smallpox would be comparable. We have begun to explore how IL-4 smallpox would spread in our county-level model on plausible, albeit uncertain, numerical assumptions—for example, that IL-4 smallpox

---

23. For the mousepox incident, see Jackson and others (2001).
24. Sharma and others (1996).

pathogenicity is twice that of smallpox, that smallpox vaccine is 50 percent as effective against IL-4 smallpox as against smallpox, and that IL-4 smallpox transmissibility equals that of smallpox. On these assumptions, containment of IL-4 smallpox is far more demanding than smallpox containment. Further research on IL-4 smallpox, and on the problem of novel pathogens in general, is planned.

It should be noted that the problem of engineered pathogens quickly raises a host of policy issues regarding the governance of scientific research in both academia and the private sector. This is another important topic for research.[25]

---

25. See Steinbruner and others (2002).

Technical Discussion

The model was written in Java, using the Ascape modeling framework (see www.brookings.edu/es/dynamics/models/ascape/main.htm). In Ascape, models consist of a variable-sized population of individual agents (objects) who coexist on a landscape of variable size and shape. In the case of this model, the landscape chosen was a two-dimensional grid resembling an overhead map. The use of an object-oriented *class* to implement Ascape agents allows for a large degree of heterogeneity among agents. Each agent object contains and updates a range of information (such as the agent's infection status, her location on the grid, and so forth). The agent decides her own actions (for example, go to work, go to the hospital, interact with another agent). Agents can be coded to have variable actions, behaviors, and data simply by creating subclasses of the basic agent type. The Ascape library of classes also provides a wide range of methods to develop interagent (and agent-landscape) interactions. In this case, the landscape was discretized into spaces corresponding to our model's major social units: homes, schools, workplaces, hospital, and morgue. Each agent has memory of where she lives, who her family members are, and where she works. The model also keeps track of all those agents with whom she has interacted over a variable length of time, which allows us to model interventions such as contact tracing.

When a run of the model begins, all agents are at home, and one agent (a commuter) has already been infected with smallpox. The model is started on day 10 of that initial agent's infection. The model proceeds in rounds: each round consists of one iteration through the entire agent population. The call order is randomized each round, and agents are processed, or activated, serially (asynchronously). On each round, when an agent is activated, she identifies her immediate neighbors (she has up to eight so-called Moore neighbors, depending on her location on the landscape) for interaction. Each interaction may, depending on a random number draw, result in a *contact*. In turn, that contact results in a transmission of the infection from the contacted agent to the active agent with probability 0 if the contacted agent is not infectious, or a positive probability (see table A-1 below) that varies according to the progress of the contacted agent's disease. Both agents record the contact in their memories, regardless of whether it resulted in a transmission (since, in reality, neither would know if transmission had in fact occurred). In the event the active agent contracts the disease, she turns green and her own internal clock of disease progression begins. After twelve days, she will turn yellow and begin infecting others.

This construction of agent interactions allows for enormous flexibility in modeling. The number of rounds each agent spends at work or school, the number of interactions each agent has per round, how often an interaction results in a contact, how often a contact results in transmission are all variable in our model and subject to sensitivity analysis. For the runs presented in this paper, each full day consists of twenty rounds, divided equally between daytime and nighttime. Thus a child spends ten rounds at home (night) and ten rounds at school (day). On each round, agent interactions proceed as discussed earlier. Note that the agent's neighbors are fixed at home (they are the same each day), whereas they are variable at work (the agent lands at the same workplace, but in a different random location at work each day).

We further make the number of contacts stochastic. Fewer contacts are assumed to occur at the workplace or school than at the home or hospital. This reflects the observation that transmission usually occurs as the result of direct contact between individuals, which is more likely to occur at home.[26] The likelihood of an interaction resulting in a contact at home is 1.0 and at work is 0.3. The model records an agent's contacts during the three days before she turns red.

To summarize, a day consists of ten rounds at home followed by ten rounds at work or school. The model tracks each individual agent's disease progression on a daily basis.

Stochasticity plays an important role in the model. Our model employs the pseudorandom number generator from the Java 2 platform. The generator uses a 48-bit seed, which is modified using a linear congruential formula.[27] By recording the random seed used in each run, we can faithfully reproduce any run generated by the model. All random events occur at the agent level; that is, the agent draws a random number from a uniform distribution and, depending on the parameter value for the event in question, the agent's

---

26. Fenner (1988).
27. See Knuth (1998), sec. 3.2.1.

state changes. The following elements of the model depend on a random draw:

—Which agent is the index case

—The order in which agents are activated

—The agent's workplace (home town, other town, hospital)

—The agent's daily location in her workplace

—Whether or not an agent is traced and/or vaccinated

—Vaccine efficacy

—Whether or not a given interaction results in a contact

—Whether or not a given contact results in a transmission

There are also various aspects of epidemics that involve delays and lags. Although we have not fully explored these areas in our model, we plan to introduce a stochastic delay in trace vaccination. The current version assumes a fixed delay of two days between the time an agent is diagnosed and when her contacts are vaccinated. In future work, this delay will be drawn from a Poisson distributed clock.

Table A-1 summarizes the model's numerical parameters. For each parameter, we list the range of possible (and plausible) values and the value assigned in the runs presented. Calibration to historical data was discussed in the text. Departures from these parameter settings are also noted in the text.

TABLE A-1. Numerical Parameters

Parameter	Chosen value	Possible range
Transmission rate per contact during regular transmission period	0.2	0–1.0
Transmission rate during high-transmission period	0.4	0–1.0
Length of noncontagious period (days)	12	0–25
Length of early rash contagious period (days)	3	0–25
Start of high-transmission period (days)	16	12–25
End of high-transmission period (days)	19	12–25
Pathogenicity	0.3	0.2–0.6 (IL-4)
Percent initially vaccinated	0	0–100
Percent hospital workers initially vaccinated	0	0–100
Vaccine efficacy	1.0	0.5–1.0
Number of agents initially infected	1	1–800
Number of adults who work in hospital	10	0–50
Hospital size	10×10	10×10–30×30
Allow hospital visitors (Boolean)	False	True, false
Percent adults who commute	10	0–100
Family stays home when first member infected (Boolean)	True	False, true
Family contact tracing (percent)	100	0–100
Work contact tracing (percent)	20	0–100
Family contacts of contacts (percent)	0	0–100
Work contacts of contacts (percent)	0	0–100
Number of days of accumulated contacts to trace	3	0–15
Number of interactions per day per agent	10	10,80
Rounds per day	10	1–50
Probability of contact per home interaction	1.0	0–100
Probability of contact per work or school interaction	0.3	0–100
Probability of contact per hospital interaction	1.0	0–100
Contact tracing maximum delay (days)	2	0–10

Current Smallpox Policy

Until 1972, immunization was required for all individuals over the age of one year in the United States. In 1972, however, the government discontinued routine vaccination because the risk of serious adverse effects outweighed the rather low risk of infection, due to high vaccine coverage and minimal exposure to smallpox. In addition, practices such as ring vaccination, which were extremely successful in the global eradication effort, further encouraged the cessation of routine smallpox vaccination.[28]

However, bioterrorism concerns have renewed interest in the creation of a substantial smallpox vaccination policy in the United States. Therefore, the Centers for Disease Control (CDC) has updated the response plans used in the 1970s. The current interim Smallpox Response Plan and Guidelines (available at: www.bt.cdc.gov/agent/smallpox/response-plan/index.asp [accessed December 10, 2002]) employs many of the methods used successfully to control outbreaks more than thirty years ago. The main concept is to control any smallpox epidemic using ring vaccination. The size of the ring of individuals may be modified according to

---

28. The term *ring vaccination* is used variously to denote different forms of targeted (as against mass) vaccination. As in the CDC's usage, it normally involves, but need not be limited to, trace vaccination.

the scale of the outbreak, the level of resources available, and the effectiveness of the method. Thus, health officials would first isolate suspected and confirmed smallpox cases. Subsequently, they would trace and vaccinate contacts of the isolated cases, as well as vaccinating the household members of the contacts.

The CDC guidelines prioritize groups for immunization as follows:

1. Face-to-face close contacts ($\leq$ 6.5 feet or 2 meters) or household contacts with smallpox patients after the onset of the patient's fever.
2. Persons exposed to the initial release of the virus (if the release was discovered during the first generation of cases and vaccination may still provide benefit).
3. Household members (without contraindications to vaccination) of contacts with smallpox patients (to protect household contacts should smallpox case contacts develop disease while under fever surveillance at home).
4. Persons involved in the direct medical care, public health evaluation, or transportation of confirmed or suspected smallpox patients.
5. Laboratory personnel involved in the collection and/or processing of clinical specimens from suspected or confirmed smallpox patients.
6. Other persons who have a high likelihood of exposure to infectious materials (for example, personnel responsible for hospital waste disposal and disinfection).
7. Personnel involved in contact tracing and vaccination, quarantine/isolation or enforcement, or law

enforcement interviews of suspected smallpox patients.

8. Persons permitted to enter any facilities designated for the evaluation, treatment, or isolation of confirmed or suspected smallpox patients (only essential personnel should be allowed to enter such facilities).

9. Persons present in a facility or conveyance with a smallpox case if fine-particle aerosol transmission was likely during the time the case was present (for example, a hemorrhagic smallpox case and/or a case with active coughing).

Additional groups with indirect contact would be considered for voluntary vaccination by the director of the CDC, as follows:

1. Public health personnel in the area involved in critical surveillance and epidemiological data analysis and reporting

2. Logistics, resource, and emergency management personnel

3. Law enforcement, fire, and other personnel involved in other nondirect patient care response support activities, such as crowd control, security, law enforcement, and firefighting and rescue operations

The Smallpox Response Plan and Guidelines is a draft document; the CDC acknowledges that it will require updates due to changes in resources. Furthermore, the immunological landscape of the United States has changed since the 1970s.

References

Anderson, Roy M., and Robert M. May. 1991. *Infectious Diseases of Humans: Dynamics and Control.* Oxford University Press. 1991.

Bailey, N. T. J. 1953. "The Total Size of a Stochastic Epidemic." *Biometrika* 40: 177.

Brian, J. L., L. Berry, Douglas Kiel, and Euell Elliott, eds. 2002. "Adaptive Agents, Intelligence, and Emergent Human Organization: Capturing Complexity through Agent-Based Modeling." Arthur Sackler Colloquia of the National Academy of Sciences. *Proceedings of the National Academy of Sciences* 99, supp. 3 (May 14).

Burke, Donald S. 1998. "Evolvability of Emerging Viruses." In *Pathology of Emerging Infections 2,* edited by A. M. Nelson and C. R. Horsburgh Jr., 1–12. Washington: ASM Press.

Burke, Donald S., Kenneth A. De Jong, John J. Grefenstette, Connie Loggia Ramsey, and Annie Wu. 1998. "Putting More Genetics into Genetic Algorithms." *Evolutionary Computation* 6: 387.

Burke, Donald S., Joshua M. Epstein, Derek A. T. Cummings, Jon I. Parker, Kenneth Cline, Ramesh M. Singa, and Shubha Chakravarty. 2004. "Individual-based Computational Modeling of Smallpox Epidemic Control Strategies." Johns Hopkins, Bloomberg School of Public Health and Brookings (January).

Epstein, Joshua M. 1997. *Nonlinear Dynamics, Mathematical Biology, and Social Science.* Reading, Mass.: Addison-Wesley.

Epstein, Joshua M., and Robert Axtell. 1996. *Growing Artificial Societies: Social Science from the Bottom Up.* M.I.T. Press.

Fenner, F., and others. 1988. *Smallpox and Its Eradication.* Geneva: World Health Organization.

Grefenstette, John J., Donald S. Burke, Kenneth A. De Jong, Connie L. Ramsey, and Annie S. Wu. 1997. "An

Evolutionary Computation Model of Emerging Virus Diseases." NCARAI Technical Report AIC-97-030.

Halloran, M. E., I. M. Longini, A. Nizam, and Y. Yang. 2002. "Containing Bioterrorist Smallpox." *Science* 298: 1428.

Henderson, D. A., T. V. Inglesby, J. G. Bartlett, M. S. Ascher, E. Eitzen, P. B. Jahrling, J. Hauer, M. Layton, J. McDade, M. T. Osterholm, T. O'Toole, G. Parker, T. Perl, P. K. Russell, and K. Tonat. 1999. "Smallpox as a Biological Weapon." *Journal of the American Medical Association* 281: 2127.

Jackson, Ronald J., and others. 2001. "Expression of Mouse Interleukin-4 by a Recombinant Ectromelia Virus Suppresses Cytolytic Lymphocyte Responses and Overcomes Genetic Resistance to Mousepox." *Journal of Virology* 75: 1205.

Kaplan, E. H., D. L. Craft, and L. M. Wein. 2002. "Emergency Response to a Smallpox Attack: The Case for Mass Vaccination." *Proceedings of the National Academy of Sciences.* 99: 10935.

Knuth, Donald E. 1998. *The Art of Computer Programming,* 3d ed. Vol. 2, *Seminumerical Algorithms.* Reading, Mass.: Addison-Wesley.

Koopman, Jim. 2002. "Controlling Smallpox." *Science* 298: 1342.

Koopman, J. S., S. E. Chick, C. P. Simon, C. S. Riolo, and G. Jacquez. 2002. "Stochastic Effects on Endemic Infection Levels of Disseminating versus Local Contacts." *Math Biosci* 180: 49.

Lane, J. M., F. L. Ruben, J. M. Neff, and J. D. Millar. 1969. "Complications of Smallpox Vaccination, 1968: National Surveillance in the United States." *New England Journal of Medicine* 281: 1201.

Mack, T. M. 1972. "Smallpox in Europe, 1950–1971." *Journal of Infectious Diseases* 125: 161.

O'Toole, T., M. Mair, and T. V. Inglesby. 2002. "Shining Light on 'Dark Winter.'" *Clinical Infectious Diseases* 34: 972.

Sharma, D. P., and others. 1996. "Interleukin-4 Mediates Downregulation of Antiviral Cytokine Expression and Cytotoxic T-Lymphocyte Responses and Exacerbates Vaccinia Virus Infection in Vivo." *Journal of Virology* 70: 7103.

Steinbruner, John, Elisa D. Harris, Nancy Gallagher, and Stacy Gunther. 2002. *Controlling Dangerous Pathogens: A Prototype Protective Oversight System.* Unpublished. University of Maryland (September).

Whittle, P. 1955. "The Outcome of a Stochastic Epidemic— A Note on Bailey's Paper." *Biometrika* 42: 116.

Index